BREAST CANCER GUIDE FOR WOMEN

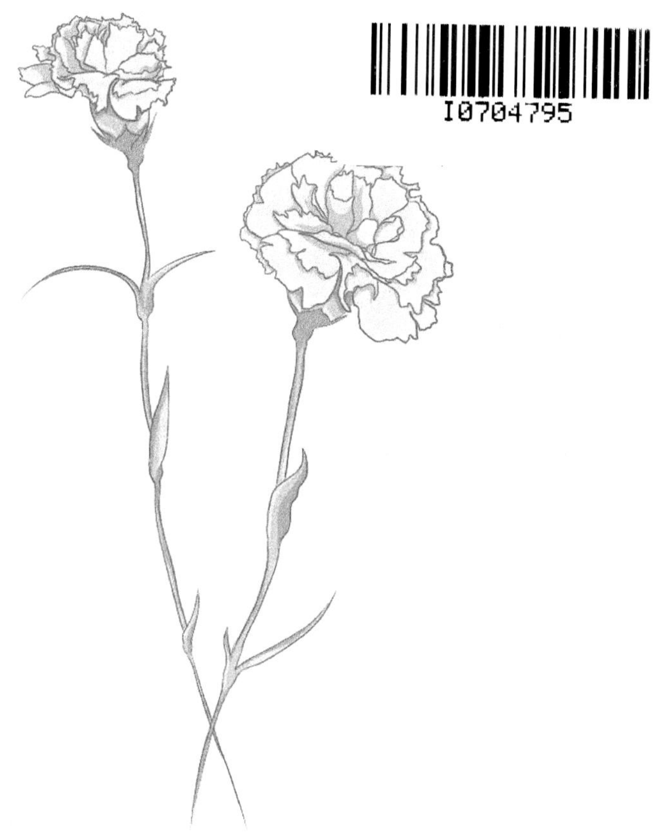

Anna Brown

A Manual for Women with Recently Diagnosed Breast Cancer

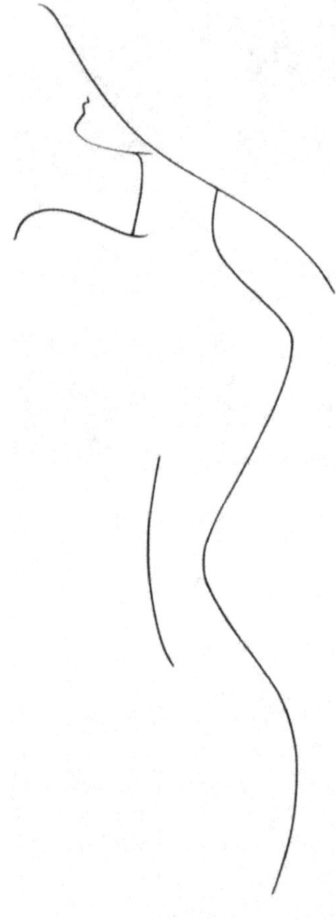

TABLE OF CONTENTS

CHAPTER ONE: INTRODUCTION

1. What is Cancer?
2. What is Breast Cancer?
3. Signs and Symptoms of Breast Cancer
4. Breast Cancer Self Examination

CHAPTER TWO: RISK FACTORS OF BREAST CANCER

1. Genetic Factors
2. Lifestyle factors

CHAPTER THREE: BREAST CANCER DIAGNOSIS

1. Getting Diagnosed
2. Embracing your Diagnosis
3. Disclosing your Breast Cancer status
   a. Telling your Kids
   b. Telling your Partner

CHAPTER FOUR: BREAST CANCER STAGES

1. Stage 0 Breast Cancer
2. Stage I Breast Cancer
3. Stage II Breast Cancer
4. Stage III Breast Cancer
5. Stage IV Breast Cancer
6. Summary

CHAPTER FIVE: BREAST CANCER TREATMENTS

1. Radiation Therapy
2. Chemotherapy
3. Hormone Therapy

CHAPTER SIX: NEED-TO-KNOW ABOUT BREAST CANCER RECURRENCE

1. Local Recurrence
2. Regional Recurrence

CHAPTER SEVEN: LIFE AFTER BREAST CANCER

CHAPTER ONE
INTRODUCTION

What is Cancer?

Cancer is a condition when a few of the body's cells grow out of control and spread to other bodily regions.

In the millions of cells that make up the human body, cancer may develop practically anywhere.

Human cells often divide (via a process known as cell growth and multiplication) to create new cells when the body requires them. New cells replace old ones when they die as a result of aging or injury.

Occasionally, this systematic process fails, causing damaged or aberrant cells to proliferate when they shouldn't. Tumors, which are tissue masses, can develop from these cells. Tumors may or may not be malignant (benign).

Cancerous tumors can move to distant parts of the body to produce new tumors, invade neighboring tissues, or both (a process called metastasis).

Malignant tumors are another name for cancerous tumors. Malignancies of the blood, including leukemias, seldom become solid tumors although many other cancers do.

Noncancerous tumors do not penetrate or spread to neighboring tissues. Benign tumors often don't come back after removal, however malignant ones can.

However, benign tumors can occasionally grow to be extremely enormous. Some, like benign brain tumors, can have grave side effects or even be fatal.

What is Breast Cancer?

One form of cancer that begins in the breast is ***breast cancer.*** It may begin in either the left or right breast. When cells start to multiply uncontrollably, cancer develops.

Although men can sometimes develop breast cancer, breast cancer affects nearly exclusively women.

It's crucial to realize that the majority of breast lumps are benign and not cancerous (malignant).

Breast tumors that are not cancerous are abnormal growths that do not spread to the exterior of the breast.

While most benign breast lumps are not life-threatening, some of them can raise a woman's chance of developing breast cancer.

Different areas of the breast might give rise to breast cancer. The lobules, ducts, nipples, connective tissues, and blood and lymph arteries are the primary components of a the breast:

1. **Lobules:** The glands that produce breast milk are called lobules. Lobular tumors are tumors that develop here.

2. **Ducts:** The milk is transported to the nipple via ducts, which are tiny channels that emerge from the lobules. The most typical area for breast cancer to begin is here. Ductal malignancies are cancers that develop here.

3. **Nipples:** The nipple is a hole in the breast's skin where the ducts combine and grow in size so that milk may escape the breast. The areola, a somewhat thicker, darker skin layer, surrounds the nipple. The nipple is

where Paget disease of the breast, a less prevalent form of breast cancer, can begin.

4. **Connective tissues:** The ducts and lobules are surrounded by fat and connective tissue (stroma), which aids in holding them in place. The stroma can be the site of the phyllodes tumor, a less frequent kind of breast cancer.

5. **Blood and lymph arteries:** Each breast also has lymphatic and blood arteries. A less frequent form of breast cancer called angiosarcoma can develop in the lining of these blood arteries.

SPREAD OF BREAST CANCER

When cancer cells enter the blood or lymphatic system and are subsequently transported to other regions of the body, breast cancer can spread.

Your body's immune system includes the lymph (or lymphatic) system.

It is a network of organs, ducts, and lymph nodes that cooperate to gather and transport clear lymph fluid through the bodily tissues and into the blood.

Lymph nodes are tiny, bean-sized glands. Immune system cells are present in the clear lymph fluid that fills the lymph veins, along with waste products and byproducts of tissue production.

To remove lymph fluid from the breast, lymph vessels are used. Cancer cells may infiltrate those lymphatic channels in the case of breast cancer and begin to proliferate in lymph nodes.

The majority of the breast's lymphatic vessels discharge into:

1. Axillary lymph nodes, which are lymph nodes under the arm

2. Internal mammary lymph nodes, which are located close to the breastbone in the chest.

3. The supraclavicular (above the collar bone) and infraclavicular (below the collar bone) lymph nodes around the collar bone.

There is a greater likelihood that cancer cells will have metastasized (moved to other places in your body) if they have already migrated to your lymph nodes.

Some women without cancer cells in their lymph nodes may later acquire metastases, while not all women with cancer cells in their lymph nodes do so.

TYPES OF BREAST CANCER

Invasive Breast Cancer

Breast cancer that has progressed into the breast tissue around it is referred to as invasive (or infiltrating). According to where they start to form in the breast, the two most prevalent kinds of invasive breast cancer are:

Invasive ductal carcinoma (IDC): The milk ducts, which are the tubes that convey milk from the lobules to the nipple, are the site of invasive ductal carcinoma (IDC), a kind of invasive breast cancer. About 80% of all cases of breast cancer are invasive ductal carcinomas, making it the most prevalent kind.

Invasive lobular carcinoma (ILC): is a kind of invasive breast cancer that begins in the lobules, or milk-producing glands of the breast. It is the second most prevalent kind of breast cancer, accounting for 10% of all invasive breast cancers.

Non-invasive Breast Cancer

Breast cancer that is non-invasive (or in situ) has not progressed outside of the original breast tissue. Precancers are another name for non-invasive breast cancers. Non-invasive breast cancer mostly comes in two forms:

Ductal carcinoma in situ (DCIS): Non-invasive breast cancer that has not moved past the milk ducts where it first appeared is known as ductal carcinoma in situ (DCIS). Although DCIS is not immediately life-threatening, it is thought to be a precursor to invasive breast cancer and raises the possibility of getting it later in life. DCIS accounts for around 16% of all breast cancer diagnoses.

Lobular carcinoma in situ (LCIS): LCIS stands for lobular carcinoma in situ, a kind of non-invasive breast cancer that has not moved past the original lobules. Despite its name, LCIS is not a genuine breast cancer; instead, it is a benign breast disease.

Signs and Symptoms of Breast Cancer

Having a breast lump is most frequently linked to breast cancer. However, depending on the particular form of breast cancer you have, your symptoms may change.

Although many breast cancer patients do experience lumps, this is not always the case. It's crucial to be aware of the additional symptoms and indicators.

The body generally emits specific warning signals. The most frequent of them is a breast lump, which can be seen anywhere from your armpit to your chest wall. Nipple bleeding or discharge, as well as associated discomfort, may be present. Your nipple may appear flattered or caved in, and there may be redness and/or swelling in any portion of the breast, in just one breast, or both breasts.

Breast changes or some of these symptoms do not always indicate breast cancer. An accurate diagnosis is based on more than simply physical symptoms.

Your breast health greatly depends on your awareness of how your breasts typically feel and appear.

Mammograms do not always detect breast cancer, despite the need for routine screening tests for the disease.

This implies that you must be aware of how your breasts typically feel and appear so that you can notice any changes.

A new lump or tumor is the most typical sign of breast cancer, even though the majority of breast lumps are benign. Although breast tumors can sometimes be soft, spherical, sensitive, or even painful, they are more likely to be cancer if they are a painless, hard mass with uneven borders.

The following are other signs of breast cancer:

1. Full or partial breast swelling (even if no lump is felt).
2. Skin dimpling (sometimes looking like an orange peel).
3. Nipple or breast pain.
4. Nipple retracting (turning inward).
5. Red, dry, flaky, or thickened nipple or breast skin.
6. Nipple discharge (other than breast milk).
7. Swollen lymph nodes in the area of the collarbone or under the arm (sometimes, this can indicate the

spread of breast cancer even before the initial tumor in the breast is large enough to be felt).

There are several benign (non-cancerous) breast disorders that can also cause similar symptoms. Nevertheless, it's crucial to get any new breast tumor, lump, or alteration examined by a skilled medical practitioner so the reason may be identified and treated, if necessary.

Keep in mind that frequent breast cancer screenings do not replace understanding what to look for.

Breast cancer may frequently be found early, before any symptoms show, thanks to screening mammography. You have a higher chance of receiving effective treatment if breast cancer is discovered early.

Breast Cancer Self Examination

Women can check their breasts step-by-step with a breast self-exam. You can spot anything that feels off by often touching and glancing at your breasts.

You can find changes that could be symptoms of infection or breast cancer by performing monthly breast self-exams (such as breast lumps or spots that feel different). Early detection of breast cancer greatly improves survival rates.

Examining oneself is crucial for breast health. However, they shouldn't take the place of the examinations and screening tests (like mammograms) advised by doctors. You ought to continue visiting your gynecologist and/or primary care physician frequently.

Every month, women should perform a breast self-exam. After their period, women who are still menstruation (have a regular period) should undertake a breast self-exam. Women can choose a day each month, even if they no longer have periods or have highly irregular ones. Pick a day that is predictable and simple to remember, such as the first or last day of the month or your favorite number.

Breast Self-exam steps:

1. **Visual assessment:** Stand in front of a mirror without your shirt or bra on. Your arms should be at your sides. Keep an eye out for any changes to the nipples, dimpling in the skin, breast swelling, or breast shape. Next, extend your arms wide in front of you while searching for the same objects. Finally, press forcefully with your hands on your hips to get your chest muscles to contract. Recheck for the same modifications. Don't forget to examine both breasts.

2. **Manual examination while standing up:** Remove your shirt and bra and use your right hand to feel your left breast before doing the same with your left. Press on each area of one breast using the pads of your three middle fingers. Apply gentle pressure first, then medium, and finally firm. Check your body for any lumps, thick areas, or other changes. You may ensure that you hit every target by using a circular pattern. Next, firmly push the tissue against the arm. Before gently squeezing the nipple to check for discharge, make sure to look under the areola. On the opposite side of your body, repeat the procedures.

3. **Examining your breasts when lying down:** Your breast tissue distributes more evenly while you're lying down. So if your breasts are big, this is an excellent posture to feel for changes. Place a cushion beneath your

right shoulder when lying down. your right arm should be behind your head. Apply the same method as in step 2 with your left hand, pressing all areas of the breast tissue and under your arm with the pads of your fingers. Last but not least, flip the pillow to the opposite side and examine the opposite breast and armpit. Before gently squeezing the nipple to check for discharge, make sure to look under the areola.

Remain calm if you discover a lump or any other concerning changes.

The majority of self-exam results do not indicate breast cancer. However, you should still contact your healthcare provider if you see any:

1. Changes to the breast's appearance, sensation, or size.

2. Changes in the nipple's appearance or sensation.
3. Skin that is dimpling or puckering.
4. A mass, a tough knot, or a thick area within the breast tissue.
5. Nipple discharge.
6. Tugging inward at the nipple or elsewhere.
7. Persistent pain in a single location.
8. Breast swelling, either in one or both.
9. Skin warmth, redness, or dark patches.

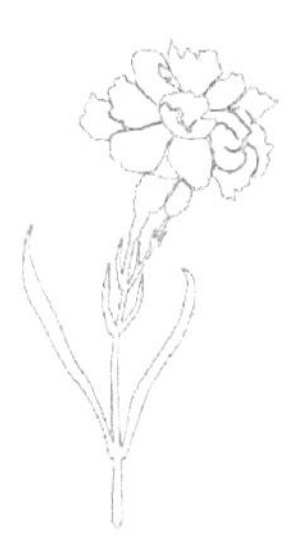

CHAPTER TWO
RISK FACTORS OF BREAST CANCER

Genetic Factors

It is believed that 5% to 10% of breast cancers are inherited and are brought on by faulty genes that are handed down from parents to children.

Chromosomes contain brief DNA (deoxyribonucleic acid) fragments known as genes. The blueprints for constructing proteins are found in DNA.

Additionally, proteins regulate the composition and operation of every cell in your body.

Consider your genes as a guide for cell development and operation. DNA alterations or faults are comparable to spelling typos. They may give the incorrect set of instructions, which would result in improper cell development or function. If a gene in any one individual contains an error, that fault will manifest itself in all the cells that carry the affected gene.

This is comparable to having an instruction manual with the same typographical error in every copy.

DNA modifications fall into two categories: those that are inherited and those that develop over time. DNA alterations that are inherited are transferred from parent to kid. Mutations or germ-line modifications are terms used to describe inherited DNA changes.

Somatic alterations are DNA mutations that take place throughout a lifetime as a result of the aging process naturally occurring or exposure to toxins in the environment. While some DNA alterations are risk-free, others might result in illness or other health problems. Mutations are DNA alterations that have a detrimental effect on health.

BRCA1 (BReast CAncer gene one) and **BRCA2** mutations are linked to the majority of hereditary instances of breast cancer (BReast CAncer gene two).

All people carry the **BRCA1** and **BRCA2** genes. The purpose of the **BRCA** genes is to maintain healthy cell growth and repair cell damage in the breast, ovarian, and other tissues.

The chance of developing breast, ovarian, and other cancers rises, however, when these genes have mutations that are handed down from one generation to the next.

Up to 10% of all breast cancers, or 1 in 10 instances, may include **BRCA1** or **BRCA2** mutations. Breast cancer is not always detected in people with **BRCA1** or **BRCA2** mutations.

Breast cancer, ovarian cancer, and other malignancies are frequently hereditarily transmitted in families of **BRCA1** or **BRCA2** mutation-positive breast cancer patients. However, the majority of those who get breast cancer have no family history of the condition, and neither did they inherit a genetic mutation connected to the disease.

If you have blood relatives (grandmothers, mothers, sisters, aunts) on either your mother's or father's side of the family who had breast cancer detected before age 50.

You are much more likely to have a genetic mutation associated with breast cancer if:

1. On the same side of the family or in the same person, there occurs ovarian and breast cancer.

2. You have a triple-negative breast cancer patient in your family.

3. In addition to breast cancer, your family also has malignancies of the prostate, melanoma, pancreas, stomach, uterus, thyroid, colon, and/or sarcoma.

4. Both breasts of women in your family have been affected by cancer.

Lifestyle factors

Personal habits including nutrition and exercise are linked to several breast cancer risk factors:

Consuming Alcohol
No doubt drinking alcohol increases the chance of developing breast cancer. According to the amount of alcohol drunk, the danger rises. Women who use one alcoholic drink per day have a little higher risk (about 7% to 10%) than those who

abstain from alcohol, while those who consume two to three drinks per day face a roughly 20% increased risk. Other cancers are also associated with an increased risk of drinking alcohol.

Being Overweight
After menopause, being overweight or obese raises the chance of developing breast cancer.

Before menopause, a woman's ovaries produce the majority of her estrogen, with adipose tissue producing the remainder. Most estrogen after menopause (when the ovaries cease producing it) originates from adipose tissue.

After menopause, having more fat tissue can enhance estrogen levels and increase the risk of developing breast cancer.

Blood insulin levels are frequently higher in overweight women. Some malignancies, particularly breast cancer, have been related to higher insulin levels.

The relationship between breast cancer risk and weight is complicated, though. For instance:

Women who put on weight as adults are at increased risk for developing breast cancer after menopause. The risk is lower for women who are overweight or obese before menopause. The causes of this are not entirely obvious.

Additionally, various forms of breast cancer may respond differently to weight. For instance:

After menopause, being overweight is more strongly associated with a higher chance of developing hormone receptor-positive breast cancer.

According to several studies, having excess body fat before menopause may raise your chance of developing less frequent triple-negative breast cancer.

Not engaging in any exercise
There is mounting evidence that regular exercise lowers the risk of breast cancer, particularly in postmenopausal women.

How much activity is required is a major concern. Even a few hours a week may be beneficial, according to some research, while more seems to be preferable.

It is unclear exactly how exercise might lower breast cancer risk, but it may be because of how it affects hormone levels, body weight, and inflammation.

Not having children
Overall, the risk of breast cancer is slightly higher in women who have never given birth or who had their first child after the age of

30. Early pregnancy and several pregnancies lower the risk of breast cancer.

The impact of pregnancy on the risk of breast cancer is complicated, though. For instance, the first ten years following having a child are when breast cancer risk is highest. then, as time passes, the danger decreases.

Use of Birth control

Hormones are used in several birth control techniques, which may raise the risk of breast cancer.

Oral contraceptives: According to the majority of studies, breast cancer risk is marginally higher for women who use oral contraceptives (birth control pills) than for those who don't. Within ten years of stopping the pills, this risk appears to return to normal.

Shots for birth control: Although not all studies have found this, some have suggested that getting shots of long-acting progesterone every three months may increase the risk of breast cancer.

Skin patches, vaginal rings, intrauterine devices (IUDs), and implants for birth control

These birth control methods also use hormones, which theoretically could promote the development of breast cancer.

Few studies have examined the relationship between the use of birth control implants, patches, and rings and the risk of breast cancer, despite some studies suggesting one between the use of hormone-releasing IUDs and the disease.

Radiation

We are surrounded by this energy from electromagnetic waves, which can be found in the ground and X-rays used in medicine. Radiation and breast cancer may be related, according to research. However, it is unclear whether radiofrequency radiation, a different low-energy form of radiation that is emitted by Bluetooth, Wi-Fi, and mobile phones, is associated with cancer.

Poor diet

A diet that is unhealthy tends to be low in whole foods, such as whole grains and fresh fruits and vegetables and high in highly processed foods, such as chips, cookies, and candy.

You could develop cancer as a result. As well as consuming a lot of processed and red meat.

High-heat cooking releases chemicals that cause cancer in the food. Limit your weekly consumption of red meat to three servings. This weighs 12 to 18 ounces altogether. According to a study, young women who consumed a lot of red meat in their teenage and early adult years had a 22% increased risk of developing breast cancer in the future.

Minimal Vitamin D

Low amounts might increase your chance of developing breast cancer. There are a few foods and pills that contain vitamin D. When sunlight is absorbed by your skin, your body produces it. It may even halt the spread of cancer.

Breast cancer claims more lives in the North-eastern United States than it does in warmer areas. But excessive exposure to the sun increases your risk of developing skin cancer.

It typically suffices to get fifteen minutes of sunshine three times each week.

CHAPTER THREE
BREAST CANCER DIAGNOSIS

Getting Diagnosed

Breast cancer is diagnosed using a variety of assays. The tests listed below may be used to find breast cancer or to check on a patient after a diagnosis:

IMAGING TESTS

Images of the interior of the body are produced during imaging exams. They can demonstrate the spread of cancer. To find out more about a worrisome spot in the breast discovered during screening, the following imaging studies of the breast may be performed. In addition to this, new test formats are also being researched.

- **Diagnostic Mammography:** In contrast to screening mammography, diagnostic mammography takes more images of the breast. When a person exhibits symptoms, such as a new lump or nipple discharge, it is frequently utilized. If a screening mammogram reveals anything worrisome, diagnostic mammography may also be used.

- **Ultrasound**: An ultrasound takes an image of the breast tissue using sound waves. An ultrasound can tell a cyst filled with fluid from a solid tumor, which is typically not cancer but may be.

- **Magnetic Resonance Imaging(MRI):** Instead of using x-rays, an MRI creates precise pictures of the body using magnetic fields. Before the scan, a special dye known as a contrast medium is administered to better visualize the potential malignancy.

The patient receives this dye through injection into a vein. After receiving a cancer diagnosis, a breast MRI may be performed to determine the extent of the illness in the breast or to screen the other breast for malignancy.

For those with a very high risk of getting breast cancer and for certain women who have a history of the disease, breast MRI may also be a screening option in addition to mammography.

If chemotherapy or endocrine therapy is administered first, followed by a second MRI for surgical planning, MRI may also be used to diagnose locally advanced breast cancer.

Finally, after breast cancer detection and therapy, MRI may be utilized as a surveillance technique.

BIOPSY

A biopsy is the removal of a tiny sample of tissue for microscopic analysis. Merely a biopsy can definitively diagnose cancer; other tests can only hint that it may be present. The material is then examined by a pathologist.

A pathologist is a medical professional who focuses on analyzing lab results and assessing cells, tissues, and organs to identify diseases.

The method and/or size of the needle used to obtain the tissue sample are used to categorize the various types of biopsies.

Biopsies by fine needle aspiration: A little sample of cells is taken during this kind of biopsy using a thin needle.

Core needle biopsy: To get a bigger tissue sample during this sort of biopsy, a broader needle is used. Typically, this is the biopsy method of choice.

Cancer biomarkers, such as hormone receptor status (ER, PR), and HER2 status, will be examined if a tumor is found to assist determine the best course of treatment.

The tumor cells have these biomarkers. Although there are other kinds of biomarkers that can be discovered in the blood or other bodily fluids, they are not frequently utilized to confirm a breast cancer diagnosis.

They are created by the tumor or the body as a defense mechanism against malignancy. The doctor will use this information to make a treatment plan recommendation.

To minimize the patient's suffering during the surgery, local anesthetic, a painkilling drug, is utilized.

Surgical biopsy: Most tissue is removed during this kind of biopsy. A surgical biopsy is typically not advised to identify breast cancer since surgery is best performed after a cancer diagnosis.

To minimize the quantity of tissue taken, non-surgical core needle biopsies are frequently advised for the diagnosis of breast cancer.

Using a needle biopsy for diagnosis lowers the number of people who have unnecessary surgery since many people who are advised to get a breast biopsy do not have cancer.

Biopsy with Image guidance: Using an imaging method, such as mammography, ultrasound, or MRI, a needle is directed to the site of the tumor or calcifications during this treatment. These can be tiny needle aspiration biopsies but are typically core needle biopsies.

A particular kind of image-guided biopsy called a stereotactic biopsy uses mammography to direct the needle. What kind of biopsy is ideal for your circumstance will be disclosed to you by your doctor.

When a breast is being biopsied, a small metal clip is typically inserted to mark the location of the biopsy sample in case the tissue turns out to be cancerous and additional surgery is required.

Since this clip is typically made of titanium, it won't interfere with any upcoming imaging tests, but check with your doctor first.

Biopsy of a Sentinel lymph node: The lymph node or group of lymph nodes that cancer first invades when it spreads through the lymphatic system is known as the "sentinel" lymph node. These are typically the axillary lymph nodes, which are lymph nodes under the arms of breast cancer.

To determine whether there is cancer in the lymph nodes close to the breast, a sentinel lymph node biopsy procedure is used.

Examination of the biopsy sample

Your doctor can learn about particular characteristics of a malignancy by analyzing the sample(s) taken during the biopsy, which can assist them to decide on your treatment options.

Characteristics of a tumor.

Determine if the tumor is invasive or non-invasive (in situ), whether it is ductal, lobular, or another kind of breast cancer, and whether cancer has spread to the lymph nodes by microscopic examination of the tumor.

The margin width—the distance from the tumor to the edge of the tissue that was removed—is assessed as well as the margins or edges of the tumor.

Progesterone Receptors (PR) and Estrogen Receptors (ER).
A patient's risk of recurrence (the risk that cancer will return) and the sort of treatment that is most likely to reduce that risk are both determined by testing for ER and PR.

The likelihood of ER-positive and/or PR-positive malignancies recurring is often decreased by hormonal therapy, commonly known as endocrine therapy or hormone-blocking therapy.

According to recommendations, everybody newly diagnosed with invasive breast cancer or when there is a breast cancer recurrence should have the ER and PR status checked on the breast tumor and/or regions of dissemination.

Testing for ER status is advised for people with ductal carcinoma in situ (DCIS) to determine whether hormone treatment can lower the risk of developing further breast cancer.

Human Epidermal Growth Factor Receptor 2 (HER2)

If medications that target the HER2 receptor, such as trastuzumab (Herceptin) and pertuzumab (Perjeta), might be able to help treat the disease, it depends on the HER2 status of the tumor.

Only aggressive tumors are subjected to this test. According to recommendations, HER2 testing should be carried out as soon as invasive breast cancer is discovered.

Additionally, testing has to be done once more on the new tumor or any regions where cancer has expanded if it has moved to another part of your body or returns after treatment.

An unambiguous positive or negative result from a HER2 test indicates whether your cancer has a high or low amount of HER2. It may be necessary to perform further testing, either on a new tumor sample or with a different test, if the findings of your test are not positive or negative.

The best course of action will need to be discussed between you and your doctor since occasionally, despite repeated testing, the results may not be conclusive.

You could be given HER2-targeted therapy as a suggested course of treatment if the malignancy is HER2-positive.

Grade.
A biopsy can also be used to identify the tumor grade. Grading describes how distinct cancer cells are from normal cells and if they seem to be developing more slowly or more quickly.

It is referred to as a "well-differentiated" or a "low-grade tumor" if the tumor contains diverse cell groupings and resembles healthy tissue in appearance. It is referred to as "poorly differentiated" or a "high-grade tumor" if the malignant tissue differs significantly from healthy tissue in appearance.

Grades 1 and 2 are both well differentiated, whereas Grade 3 is somewhat differentiated (poorly differentiated).

BLOOD TESTS

A variety of blood tests may also be required, according to your doctor. You can do these tests either before or after surgery.

Thorough blood count: The quantity of various cell types, including red blood cells and white blood cells, in a sample of a person's blood, is determined by a complete blood count (CBC). It is done to check if your bone marrow is working properly.

Blood composition: The effectiveness of your liver and kidneys is assessed by this test.

Test for hepatitis: These tests may occasionally be performed to look for signs of past hepatitis B and/or hepatitis C exposure.

Before receiving chemotherapy, you might need to take a particular drug to suppress the virus if you have signs of an active hepatitis B infection. Without this drug, chemotherapy may promote the virus' growth and liver damage. Before starting treatment, find out more about hepatitis B testing.

Your doctor will discuss the findings with you when the diagnostic tests are finished. These findings aid the clinician in describing the malignancy if it is determined to be cancer. Staging describes this.

Additional imaging studies may be advised based on cancer's stage and the tumor's biomarkers. You might require a biopsy of another place of the body to determine whether a suspicious spot detected outside of the breast and adjacent lymph nodes is cancerous.

Embracing your Diagnosis

One of the most upsetting experiences a woman may have is learning she has breast cancer. Additionally, women might not know how to get assistance.

Even after the immediate shock of a diagnosis has subsided, distress generally persists. Women may encounter additional issues when they start what is frequently a protracted treatment procedure.

For instance, they can discover that their connections are in disarray. They could experience constant fatigue. They could be extremely concerned about their symptoms, medical care, and eventual death. They can encounter prejudice from employers or insurance providers.

These kinds of elements can have a role in long-term stress, anxiety, and depressive symptoms.

You could feel as though you no longer have control over your life after learning you have breast cancer. The choices you must make might be too much for you to handle. These emotions are typical.

However, don't allow them to stop you from acting. Learn as much as you can about breast cancer initially. Learn about available therapies, side effects, and clinical studies. Always keep in mind that while doctors can offer possibilities, the final choice should be made together.

Another method to feel in control is to **know what to anticipate.** Maintaining as regular of a schedule as you can also be beneficial.

Be tolerant. Breast cancer treatment takes patience, acceptance, a strong will, and support. Numerous others also find courage in their spirituality and religious beliefs.

One of the finest things you can do is to **speak with your doctor.** Be honest with one another. You'll develop confidence and trust as a result of this. Making important treatment decisions as a team will also be made easier with its assistance.

Perhaps the worst thing that could ever happen to you is being diagnosed with breast cancer. Nevertheless, you might be able to take away some positives. Many breast cancer survivors claim that their social networks and outlook on life have improved as a result of their diagnosis.

Others have forged new bonds, reconnected with old ones, and discovered power inside themselves that they were unaware they possessed.

As a result, many individuals now offer support to those dealing with breast cancer. **You can decide that you can also inform and assist other people who are dealing with breast cancer.**

Any breast cancer treatment aims to eradicate the disease and provide patients with the greatest chance of surviving.

Even the most effective therapies have negative consequences; hot flushes, hair loss, and exhaustion are typical side effects.

Body image changes can result from changes in physical characteristics. Stress and worry may result from this. A mastectomy may be quite challenging. Reconstruction and prosthesis are two options that may assist with body image issues.

You might want assistance with daily errands or housework while undergoing treatment.

Never be embarrassed to seek assistance. Ask for assistance with child care and grocery shopping. Additionally, you could require transportation to and from your medical visits. Be specific about what you require. It will raise your chances of receiving the assistance you require.

Disclosing your Breast Cancer status

It can be quite challenging to inform family and friends that you have breast cancer, and you might worry about their reaction.

You may be still processing your diagnosis. You could worry about how and when to inform them, as well as about the questions they might have. However, being honest with others about your cancer may make it easier for them to support you and help you deal.

When informing people, having an informed friend or family member at your side might help.

Starting with the fundamentals of your diagnosis and available treatments might be beneficial before letting the conversation flow organically from there. It's possible that you don't want to provide specifics or that you're still learning a lot yourself. You might provide folks with written material if you don't want to or are unable to go into great depth at first.

Different people respond differently to unfavorable news. What they say might differ depending on:

- Their proximity to you.
- Whether they anticipated it.
- Their own experience with cancer and other catastrophic diseases.

Others may find it difficult to process it, while others may feel uneasy or anxious.

Most people associate the word "cancer" negatively, and they may unintentionally respond insensitively as a result. People frequently speak inappropriately when they are feeling stressed, scared, or helpless.

In addition, it may seem as though others are reluctant to discuss your disease with you although they may only be reluctant to disturb you.

Some individuals could be "overly optimistic" to uplift your spirits in the wake of your diagnosis. They could use expressions like "battling your condition" and "fighting cancer." This may give you the impression that you should be in charge of your circumstances and that any setbacks are your fault. It could also give you the impression that you must have a "stiff upper lip" and refrain from having any "bad" days.

Talking to others about how you're feeling could be helpful; if you find their comments to be harsh or insensitive, having a conversation with them about how you perceive your breast cancer might help. It may be quite beneficial to talk about your sentiments with those closest to you and let them know how they can support you.

Everyone handles unpleasant news in various ways.

Avoid feeling as though you must conceal your emotions or put on a strong front for the benefit of others since this can seem like an added weight.

If you have kids, one of the hardest things you'll have to do is inform them you have breast cancer.

It's always preferable to be upfront since kids might get even more anxious if they think anything is being kept from them. Even if you are the person who knows your child the best, it may be incredibly challenging to know what to say to them.

TELLING YOUR KIDS

There is no simple way to inform your children that you have cancer, however, there are a few things to consider:

1. Prepare in advance.
Although you don't need to have a prepared speech, you should have a general idea of what you want to say and prepared responses to any questions they could have.

For instance, they could inquire as to what cancer is in general and how it would affect your day-to-day activities.

2. Pay attention to the good.
Even though you might feel overwhelmed and worried about the future, do your best to remain upbeat for your children. Tell them, for instance, that you are receiving the greatest treatment available. Let them know that the breast cancer survival rate is encouraging.

You aim to provide them comfort without making any promises about what the future may bring.

3. Deliver truthful, understandable information.

Children have excellent intuition and often pay more attention than they realize. Withholding information that clarifies your diagnosis might lead them to terrifying assumptions.

Don't saturate them with the knowledge they can't comprehend. It's enough to have an overview of what's going on. Give frank, age-appropriate explanations of the illness, its management, and any potential physical and psychological impacts it may have on you.

4. Put your diagnosis into context.

Young children frequently have false beliefs about your illness. For instance, they could believe that what they did cause your illness. Tell them you're not to fault for getting cancer.

It's also possible that they believe your cancer is spreadable, much like a cold. They could believe that if they go too near to you, they'll get it. Spend some time explaining how cancer develops and how embracing you won't harm them.

5. Let them know they'll never be forgotten.

Young children want regularity and assurance during stressful situations. Even if you might not have the time or energy to give them ongoing care, reassure them that they will receive the necessary help.

Give them specifics on who will be handling things for them if you are unable to.

6. Describe the new standard.

Even while you might not have time to coach the soccer team or accompany students on field excursions, you'll still find time to be with your kids. Give examples of particular activities you can do together, like reading or watching TV.

7. Describe the possible physical effects of cancer therapy on you.

Inform them that you are receiving aggressive cancer treatment and that you will probably change the way you look and feel. Inform them that you could shed several pounds.

Other potential symptoms include hair loss, extreme fatigue, and occasional illness. Tell them that even if things have changed, you are still their parent.

8. Get them ready for your mood changes.

Inform them that you are not feeling sad or angry because of anything they did. No matter how difficult things become, make sure they know you love them and aren't angry with them.

9. Allow them to ask questions

There will probably be questions from your children, some of which you may not have thought to ask. Give them the chance to ask any questions they may have. Give a sincere and acceptable response.

They may feel more at ease and less unclear about what it means to have a parent with cancer as a result of this.

TELLING YOUR PARTNER

For every relationship to be successful, there must be open communication. Whether you're talking about your health, sex, or money issues, it's crucial to be open and honest with each other. You must pay special attention as well.

Keep in mind that your spouse will probably feel just as shocked and terrified to learn about your disease as you were.

Allow them some time to acclimate.

Inform them of your needs at this time. Tell your spouse that you want them to take an active role in your therapy. Make it clear whether you prefer to handle things yourself.

Talk to your spouse about their needs as well. They could be worried about your capacity to carry out your share of domestic duties.

When you know you won't be able to handle tasks like cooking or grocery shopping on your own, try to come up with solutions with your spouse while still being considerate of their needs.

Allowing your partner to accompany you to a doctor's visit is preferable. They will better comprehend what is ahead if they have greater knowledge about your cancer and its therapies.

Set aside sometime each week for the two of you to sit and speak. Whatever feelings surface, from rage to annoyance, you should feel free to express them. Consider seeing a couples counselor or therapist if your partner doesn't understand your condition or can't manage it.

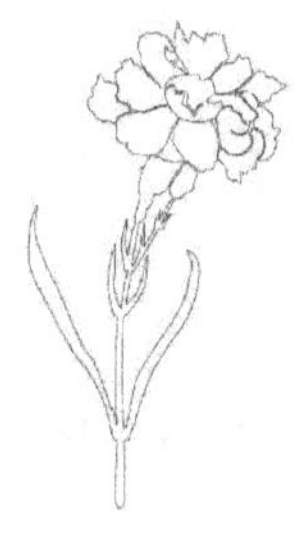

CHAPTER FOUR
BREAST CANCER STAGES

A breast cancer's stage may be determined by the size of the tumor, whether it has spread to nearby lymph nodes if it has reached distant regions of the body, and what cancer's biomarkers are.

Staging can be carried out either before or following surgery on a patient. The pathologic stage refers to staging performed after surgery, whereas the clinical stage refers to staging performed before surgery.

The stage of the cancer is determined by diagnostic testing, therefore staging may not be complete until all of the tests have been completed.

Knowing the stage aids the doctor in recommending the best course of action and can assist in determining the prognosis, or likelihood of recovery, for a patient.

Doctors use the following three aspects to identify the stage of breast cancer:

- **T,** the breast tumor's size.
- **N,** the number of lymph nodes afflicted and the extent to which the malignancy has spread.
- **M,** metastasis, if cancer has spread to different parts of the body.

Stage 0 Breast Cancer

You now have a lot of questions after the doctor informed you that your breast cancer is at stage 0. Why does that matter? Is cancer even present?

In actuality, medical professionals are not sure as well. It is regarded as the first stage of breast cancer by some doctors. Some people view it as a kind of early-stage of cancer.

Cancer is a category of illnesses characterized by aberrant cells that proliferate uncontrollably. These cells can enter neighboring tissues.

Breast cancer at stage 0 is noninvasive, meaning it has not moved to other regions of the breast or other organs from where it first appeared.

Breast cancer in stage 0 often has no further symptoms. Stage 0 breast cancer can occasionally be found by mistake by a clinician, for example, following a biopsy or while doing an imaging test on a separate lump.

Some patients may be diagnosed by doctors following a routine screening or after detecting a lump.

Cancer that has metastasized has spread to additional organs. Even when stage 0 breast cancer has not spread, a patient can still need therapy to stop metastasis in the future.

Depending on the sort of stage 0 breast cancer a person has, as well as other variables like age and family history, a person can either receive the best therapy or not.

Stage 0 breast cancer comes in two different varieties:

Lobular Carcinoma In Situ(LCIS)
Breast milk-producing gland cancer is referred to as lobular carcinoma. The term "lobes" or "lobules" refers to these glands.

The lobular cancer stage known as lobular carcinoma in situ (LCIS) typically does not spread. It does, however, raise the possibility of getting other forms of breast cancer. Most lobular carcinoma cases in women occur between the ages of 40 and 50, just before menopause.

After menopause, this kind of cancer affects less than 1 in 10 women.

Because of this, receiving a diagnosis of LCIS may indicate that a woman may require future breast cancer tests more often.

Ductal Carcinoma In Situ(DCIS)

Breast cancer of the milk ducts is known as ductal carcinoma in situ (DCIS). Milk travels through the milk ducts, which are tubes, from the milk glands to the nipple.

DCIS has the potential to expand and worsen if left untreated. DCIS has a 50 percent chance of developing into aggressive malignancy.

Usually, LCIS won't spread to other places. However, because it increases the chance of developing additional breast cancers, it has to be carefully and frequently monitored.

Which DCIS presentations will expand and become more aggressive is impossible for doctors to anticipate.

Low-grade tumors, or those with distinct borders and modest development, may, nevertheless, have a lower propensity to spread and become invasive.

Usually, DCIS breast cancers in the very early stages don't show any symptoms.

Although it's occasionally possible to feel a little, hard lump, routine mammography screenings are how most women learn they have stage 0 breast cancer.

Stage I Breast Cancer

The earliest stage of invasive breast cancer is stage 1 disease. It has a future that is promising if treated.

The early detection of stage 1 breast cancer is greatly aided by routine breast cancer screening. As with most cancers, the better the prognosis is likely to be the earlier stage 1 breast cancer is found and treated.

Based on the tumor's size and lymph node spread, experts classify it into stages 1A and 1B.

Stage IA
A malignancy that is at stage 1A is less than 2 centimeters (cm) in size and has not spread outside the breast.

Stage IB
In lymph nodes around the breast, stage 1B breast cancer cells are present in tiny regions, and it also implies that:

No breast tumor is discovered or the breast tumor is 2 cm or less in size.

In the TNM staging classification, stage 1A breast cancer is the same as:
- T1 N0 M0

The equivalent of Stage 1B is:
- T0 N1mi M0
- T1 N1mi M0.

The **TNM** staging system stands for Tumour, Node, Metastasis.

Stage I breast cancer symptoms

Stage 1 breast cancer symptoms might include:

1. Nipple discharge
2. Skin sagging or dimples
3. Breast swelling or erythema
4. A breast bulge or an armpit bump

5. Alterations to the breast's skin's texture
6. Nipple inversion or flattening

Stage II Breast Cancer

Breast cancer that has reached stage II has spread to adjacent lymph nodes, the breast, or both. It is breast cancer in its early stages.

Cancer stage reveals its size and the extent of its dissemination. It aids your doctor in determining the best course of action.

Breast cancer staging is an extremely intricate process. Here is a condensed explanation. Before physicians can certify your final stage, several distinct elements are taken into account.

For instance, they examine a piece of your cancer to check for:

- Hormone receptors for women (estrogen and progesterone).
- The grade of your cancer's HER2 status (human epidermal growth factor receptor 2).

Stage II breast cancer may be divided into stage IIA and stage IIB.

Stage IIA

Stage IIA denotes one of the following:

- No tumor or a tumor 2 centimeters (cm) or less has been identified in the breast, and 1 to 3 armpit lymph nodes or lymph nodes close to the breastbone have been confirmed to have cancer cells.
- There is no malignancy in the lymph nodes, and the tumor is greater than 2 cm but not more than 5 cm.

Stage IIB

Denotes one of the following:

- There are little patches of cancerous cells in the lymph nodes, and the tumor is greater than 2 cm but not bigger than 5 cm.

- Cancer has progressed to one to three lymph nodes in the armpit or to the lymph nodes close to the breastbone, and the tumor is greater than 2 cm but not larger than 5 cm.

- Despite being greater than 5 cm, the tumor has not yet migrated to the lymph nodes.

Stage II Breast Cancer symptoms

Stage II breast cancer patients may not exhibit any symptoms, and the disease may only be identified during regular mammography. Stage II breast cancer signs and symptoms might include:

1. A breast or underarm bump.
2. Nipple discharge.

3. Breast skin that has creases.
4. Redness or swelling.
5. A flattened or inverted nipple.
6. Alterations to the breast skin.
7. Alterations in breast size or form.
8. Pain.

Stage III Breast Cancer

Stage 3 indicates that cancer has migrated from the breast to nearby lymph nodes, the breast's surface, or the chest wall. Additionally, it is known as locally advanced breast cancer.

To be sure cancer has not spread to other bodily areas, you could also get a CT scan.

Three categories of stage 3 breast cancer are recognized:

Stage IIIA
One of the following describes Stage 3A:

- Cancer is discovered in 4 to 9 lymph glands under the arm, or in the lymph glands close to the breastbone, but no tumor is seen in the breast, and the tumor may be of any size.

- Small clusters of breast cancer cells are seen in the lymph nodes when the tumor is greater than 5 cm.

- The tumor is larger than 5 cm and has reached up to 3 armpit lymph nodes or lymph nodes close to the breastbone.

Stage IIIB

Stage 3B indicates that the tumor has metastasized to the chest wall or the skin of the breast.

The components that surround and shield the lungs, such as the ribs, muscles, skin, or connective tissues, are referred to as the chest wall. The malignancy has produced swelling or a breakdown of the skin (ulcer).

Up to 9 armpit lymph nodes or the lymph nodes close to the breastbone may have received cancer's spread. Inflammatory breast cancer may be cancer that has spread to the breast's skin.

Stage IIIC
In stage 3C, there may or may not be a tumor, depending on its size.

However, there is cancer in the skin of the breast that has gone to the chest wall and is causing edema or ulcers.

Additionally, it has affected one or more of the following areas:

1. 10 or more lymph nodes in the armpit.
2. Lymph nodes in the armpit and close to the breastbone.

3. Lymph nodes above or below the collarbone.

Stage III Breast Cancer symptoms

Stage 3 breast cancer symptoms might include:

1. Alterations to the breast's skin, such as dimples, color changes, scaliness, or open sores.
2. A breast lump or armpit enlargement.
3. Nipple alterations such as an inverted or flattened nipple, a discharge (which can be clear or opaque, red, yellow, or green), peeling or flaking.
4. Alterations in breast size or form.
5. Discomfort, irritability, or itching.
6. Red, heated to the touch, or swollen breasts.

Stage IV Breast Cancer

Breast cancer that has reached stage 4 has spread to other bodily organs.

Other names for it include metastatic breast cancer, advanced cancer, and secondary breast cancer.

Cancer stage reveals its size and the extent of its dissemination. It aids your doctor in determining the best course of action.

In stage IV cancer:

- Any tumor size may exist.
- There may or may not be cancer cells in the lymph nodes.
- Cancer has metastasized, or spread, to the bones, lungs, liver, or brain, among other bodily organs.

Depending on where the disease has spread, the symptoms of metastatic breast cancer might vary greatly, however they may include:

- Difficulties peeing (either incontinence or not being able to go), which might be an indication that cancer is pressing on your back's nerves.
- Back, bone, or joint discomfort that does not go away.
- Weakness or numbness over your whole body.
- continuous dry cough.
- Respiratory issues or lack of breath.
- Chest ache.
- Reduced appetite.
- Abdominal discomfort, pain, or swelling.
- Persistent diarrhea, vomiting or losing weight.
- Jaundice (a yellow tinge to the skin and whites of your eyes).
- Severe headaches and difficulty seeing.

- Seizures.
- Decline in balance.
- Confusion.

Summary

Stage 0: This is the initial cancer warning indication. Although they haven't spread and can't yet be positively identified as cancerous, the region may contain abnormal cells.

Stage I: The earliest stage of breast cancer is stage 1. Although there may be a few little cancer clusters in the lymph nodes, the tumor is only 2 cm in size.

Stage II: This denotes the beginning of cancer's spread. The breast tumor may be greater than 2 cm in size or the malignancy may have spread to many lymph nodes.

Stage III: This is regarded by doctors as a more advanced stage of breast cancer. Large or tiny, the breast tumor may have progressed to the chest and/or several lymph nodes.

In other cases, cancer has spread to the breast's skin, resulting in inflammation or skin ulcers.

Stage IV: The disease has moved beyond the breast and into other bodily parts.

CHAPTER FIVE

BREAST CANCER TREATMENTS

Your cancer location, size, whether it has spread to other parts of your body, and overall health will all affect how you are treated.

The optimum course of treatment and care for you is determined by a group of doctors and other experts.

Radiation Therapy

High doses of radiation are used in radiation treatment to either kill cancer cells or stop them from proliferating, dividing, or spreading to other organs.

There is minimal harm to neighboring healthy cells since it just affects the cancer cells.

RADIATION THERAPY TYPES

- **External Beam Radiation Therapy:** The most popular radiation therapy for breast cancer is external beam radiotherapy.

  Equipment outside of your body directs a radiation beam to the diseased spot.

- **Proton Therapy:** With proton treatment, just your breast tissue receives precisely focused radiation, not your heart or lungs.

- **Brachytherapy**: Uses an implant in your body to administer radiation to cancer.

EXTERNAL BEAM RADIATION

To provide a map for the medical team treating you, tiny markings and stickers will be applied to your skin along the treatment region.

The therapist will re-mark these areas as necessary; do not attempt to wipe them off or touch them up if they fade.

Your therapist will accompany you to the treatment room and assist you in finding the proper posture. They will then go and begin the therapy.

It's crucial to remain motionless and at ease. The therapist can see you and hear you thanks to cameras and an intercom.

If there is something that concerns you, tell them immediately away.

To adjust the equipment and your body, the therapist will come in and out of the room. You won't be touched by the machine, and the procedure won't hurt.

External beam radiation side effects

You could experience them throughout therapy, depending on the type and dose:

1. Sensitive, swollen, red, and warm skin, you could think you have a sunburn. It could peel or get soft and wet.
2. Where you were treated, you could become less sweaty.
3. Hair loss.
4. Fatigue.
5. Breast enlargement.
6. Alterations in skin sensitivity.

After your final treatment, these side effects typically subside gradually over the next 4 to 6 weeks. If you see skin changes outside the treated region, tell your doctor or nurse.

After therapy, long-term adverse effects may persist for more than a year. They may consist of:

1. A very minor skin darkening.
2. Breast pores that are enlarged.
3. Skin that is more or less sensitive.
4. Breast tissue or skin thickening
5. A change in your breast size.

The following issues are very uncommon:
1. Damaged ribs.
2. Heart injury.
3. Lungs that are inflamed.
4. If you have your lymph nodes removed, you may get lymphedema (arm swelling).
5. More cancers or tumors.
6. Aching chest wall.

UNDERSTANDING SKIN REACTIONS
These actions will assist:

1. Wash the affected area gently with warm water and mild soap. Avoid rubbing your skin. Use a soft cloth to

gently pat it dry or a cold setting on your hair dryer.

2. Avoid rubbing or scratching the treated area. If you must shave there, only use an electric razor. Don't use bandages or medical tape.

3. If your doctor or nurse hasn't recommended an ointment, cream, lotion, or powder, don't use it on the affected region. This covers deodorants, shaving creams, fragrances, and cosmetics.

4. Choose loose-fitting apparel or rough materials like wool or corduroy over garments composed of natural fibers like cotton.

5. Where you have received radiation, stay away from intense heat or cold; don't use electric heating pads, hot water bottles, or ice packs.

6. Avoid tanning beds and hot baths as well.

7. Even after your treatment is over, avoid being in the sun, especially between the hours of 10 a.m. and 2 p.m. Sun exposure can exacerbate skin conditions and result in a painful sunburn. Select sunscreen with an SPF of 30 or higher. Put on protective clothes, including a long-sleeved shirt, slacks, and a hat with a broad brim.

PROTON THERAPY

This kind of external beam radiation damages cancer cells' DNA, preventing them from proliferating or dividing, by harnessing the energy of positively charged particles called protons. You often receive it 4 to 6 weeks following surgery or chemotherapy, and for several weeks, you will have it five days a week for 30 to 45 minutes each time.

Both proton therapy and conventional cancer radiation therapy work by damaging the DNA of cancer cells to eradicate tumors.

Photons are high-energy light waves that are used in standard radiation (X-ray) to accomplish this. Radiation from X-rays is dispersed throughout your body as they pass through you.

When they reach your tumor, they continue moving. Beyond the treatment area, they continue to move. That might damage the body's healthy tissue.

Cancer is killed with proton therapy, which employs protons as charged particle beams. The majority of the protons' energy for battling cancer is directed at the tumor. They also stay within the designated perimeter. This means that any tissue close to the tumor is less likely to suffer radiation damage.

Proton treatment also offers the following advantages:

1. It's not painful.
2. It isn't intrusive (no cuts or incisions are needed).
3. It is compatible with various cancer therapies.
4. If you have breast implants, you can still utilize them.

Proton treatment has very little or no negative effects. Compared to conventional radiation therapy, people appear to take this form of radiation treatment better.

BRACHYTHERAPY
In the breast, close to the tumor, tiny radioactive seeds or pellets the size of rice grains are inserted. The size, location, and other factors of your tumor will determine if this treatment is appropriate for you.

External beam radiation or brachytherapy can be combined.

Brachytherapy Side Effects
Most individuals respond in ways like:

1. Pain
2. Bruising and
3. Redness

Problems that are less probable but conceivable include:

1. Infection.
2. Damage to the breast's fatty tissue.
3. Rib weakness and fractures are unusual events.
4. A buildup of fluid in the breast (seroma).

Chemotherapy

Drugs are used in chemotherapy to target and kill breast cancer cells. Typically, these medications are administered orally as tablets or by needle injection into a vein.

Chemotherapy is commonly used in conjunction with other therapies for breast cancer, such as surgery, radiation, or hormone therapy.

Chemotherapy can be used to treat cancer symptoms, lower the likelihood that the disease will come back, improve survival time and quality of life for cancer patients, and enhance the likelihood of a cure.

Chemotherapy may be able to manage breast cancer if it has returned or expanded, extending your life.

Or it might aid in reducing the symptoms that cancer is producing.

The adverse effects of chemotherapy for breast cancer can range from moderate and transient to severe and long-lasting. You can get advice from your doctor on whether chemotherapy is an appropriate option for you if you have breast cancer.

In the following circumstances, chemotherapy for breast cancer may be administered:

Chemotherapy following breast cancer surgery

Your doctor may advise chemotherapy to eliminate any cancer cells that were missed during surgery to remove the breast cancer and lower your chance of the disease returning. The term "adjuvant chemotherapy" refers to this.

Even if there is no sign of cancer after surgery, your doctor may advise adjuvant chemotherapy if you have a high chance of cancer coming back or metastasizing (spreading to other areas of your body). If cancer cells are discovered in lymph nodes close to the afflicted breast, you might be at an increased risk of metastasis.

Chemotherapy before Breast Cancer Surgery

To reduce bigger malignancies, chemotherapy may occasionally be administered before surgery (also known as neoadjuvant treatment or preoperative chemotherapy). This might:

1. Give the surgeon the greatest opportunity to thoroughly remove the malignancy.

2. Allow the surgeon to merely remove cancer as opposed to the whole breast.

3. Reduce the severity of the illness in the lymph nodes to enable less invasive surgery for the nodes

4. Reduce the likelihood that cancer will recur.

5. Help your doctor choose which chemotherapy drugs are best for you based on how well your cancer reacts to treatment. This will help them determine your prognosis.

Neoadjuvant treatment is frequently employed in:
1. Aggressive breast cancer.
2. Breast cancer that is HER2-positive.
3. High-stage breast cancers.
4. Lymph nodes that have been affected by cancer.
5. Bigger breast tumors.

Chemotherapy might be used as the main treatment if your breast cancer has spread to other areas of your body and surgery is not an option.

Targeted treatment may be used in conjunction with it.

Chemotherapy for advanced breast cancer often aims to extend and enhance the quality of life rather than to treat the illness.

Risks

Drugs used in chemotherapy circulate throughout the body. The medications you take and how you react to them will affect any side effects. The severity of side effects may worsen as the treatment progresses. The majority of adverse effects are transient and go away after therapy. Chemotherapy occasionally has lasting or irreversible consequences.

Short-term side effects

Chemotherapy medications, which target rapidly proliferating cancer cells, can also harm rapidly proliferating healthy cells, including those in the bone marrow, digestive system, and hair follicles.

After the course of treatment is complete or within a year of finishing chemotherapy, these side effects frequently fade away. They could last for a while in certain instances.

Typical immediate side effects include:
1. Hair loss
2. Fatigue
3. Appetite loss
4. Nausea and diarrhea
5. Bloating or diarrhea
6. Oral sores
7. Skin and nail modifications
8. Increased chance of contracting an illness (due to fewer white blood cells that help fight infection).
9. Nerve injury (neuropathy).
10. Memory and attention issues caused by cognitive dysfunction commonly referred to as "chemo brain".

Long-term side effects

Some breast cancer chemotherapy medications can have long-term negative effects, such as:

1. **Infertility**: Infertility is one potential adverse effect that could persist. Some anticancer medications cause ovarian damage.

   Menopause symptoms like hot flashes and dry vaginal discharge might result from this.

   Periods of menstruation may halt or become irregular (amenorrhea). It becomes impossible to get pregnant if ovulation stops.

   Chemotherapy may cause early, irreversible menopause depending on your age. Talk to your doctor about the possibility of experiencing irreversible menopause and its effects.

Even while receiving therapy or after it is finished, you may still be able to become pregnant if you continue to menstruate. But before starting treatment, discuss with your doctor the best forms of birth control as the effects of chemotherapy are harmful to the baby.

2. **Thinned bones:** Chemotherapy-induced early menopause may increase the risk of osteopenia and osteoporosis in the women who experience it.

   These women should typically undergo routine bone density exams and, if necessary, treatments to stop further bone loss.

3. **Heart injury:** There is a very small chance that chemotherapy will weaken the heart muscle and result in other

heart issues. Future cardiac issues are more likely when certain chemotherapy drugs are used.

4. **Leukemia:** Rarely, chemotherapy for breast cancer can lead to a secondary cancer years after the chemotherapy is finished, such as leukemia, a cancer of the blood cells.

When and how often to get chemotherapy treatments
Breast cancer chemotherapy is administered in cycles. Chemotherapy cycles might range from once every week to once every three weeks. A time of recuperation follows each therapy session.

Typically, chemotherapy treatments for early-stage breast cancer last three to six months, but your doctor will modify the length of time based on your specific needs. If your breast cancer has progressed, your therapy may last longer.

Radiation treatment is often administered after chemotherapy if you have early-stage breast cancer and are also scheduled for it.

How chemotherapy is administered
Chemotherapy medications can be administered in several different ways, including tablets that you take at home.

They are often injected into a vein (IV). This is accomplished by:

1. A catheter (IV needle and tubing) in your hand or wrist.

2. A catheter port that is surgically inserted into your chest before chemotherapy. It is not necessary to locate a suitable vein at each treatment session because this port remains in place during your chemotherapy.

Typical chemotherapy treatments
Although no two chemotherapy treatments
are the same, a session can go as follows:

1. You provide a blood sample so that it
   may be used for a blood count and
   another testing.

2. You see your doctor discuss the
   findings of your blood test and discuss
   your general health.

3. Your physician makes the
   chemotherapy order.

4. You have a meeting with the medical
   professional in charge of your
   chemotherapy.

5. A quick physical examination is
   performed to measure your blood
   pressure, pulse, and temperature.

6. The IV catheter has been placed in you.

7. To avoid unpleasant side effects like nausea, anxiety, or inflammation, you take drugs.

8. The chemotherapy medications are given to you. This might need many hours.

Following a chemotherapeutic treatment

After receiving chemotherapy, you could:

1. Remove the temporary IV catheter.
2. Check the health of your vital signs.
3. Talk to your doctor about the negative effects.
4. Obtain prescriptions for home-use drugs to deal with adverse effects.
5. Don't forget to eat and drink responsibly.

6. Get guidance on how to handle body fluids such as urine, feces, vomit, semen, and vaginal secretions properly, as they may carry certain chemotherapy medications over the following 48 hours. Simply flushing the toilet twice after use can do this.

Following chemotherapy treatment, some patients feel well and may resume their routines and hobbies. Some people can experience adverse effects sooner.

At least for the first few sessions, until you see how you feel, you might want to make arrangements for someone to transport you home afterward.

Throughout the chemotherapy process
After a few sessions, you could be able to anticipate when you'll feel well and when

you might need to reduce your activity level more precisely.

You can track your general response to chemotherapy treatments and make plans for activities appropriately by marking your calendar or keeping a notebook.

The best method to maximize the benefits of chemotherapy is to strictly adhere to your treatment plan. Consult your doctor if side effects start to annoy you.

He or she might be able to change the kind or dosage of chemotherapy medicine you're taking or give you a prescription for another drug to aid with symptoms like nausea.

Your doctor may suspend chemotherapy treatment if the quantity of white blood cells in your blood falls until the white blood cell count stabilizes.

Stress reduction may be aided by relaxation practices like meditation and deep breathing.

Exercise has also been demonstrated to alleviate chemotherapy-related weariness and aid in better sleep.

Hair loss can be hidden by using hats, turbans, or wigs.

Results
Your doctor will arrange follow-up appointments after your chemotherapy treatment is finished to check for cancer recurrence and monitor for long-term adverse effects.

Expect to see a doctor every few months, then less frequently as time goes on if you don't have cancer.

Hormone Therapy

Hormonally sensitive breast cancers can be treated with hormone therapy. The two main methods of hormone therapy for breast cancer are blocking hormones from attaching to cancer cell receptors and reducing the body's hormone production.

Only breast cancers that have been found to have estrogen or progesterone receptors are treated with hormone therapy.

After surgery, hormone therapy for breast cancer is frequently used to lower the likelihood that cancer will come back.

To increase the likelihood that cancer will be completely removed during surgery, hormone therapy for breast cancer may also be used to reduce a tumor before surgery.

Hormone therapy for breast cancer may aid in controlling the disease if it has spread to other organs.

WHY IT IS DONE

Only hormone-sensitive malignancies are treated with hormone treatment for breast cancer (hormone receptor-positive breast cancers).

These malignancies are known as progesterone receptor-positive (PR positive) or estrogen receptor-positive (ER-positive) by physicians (PR positive).

This indicates that the natural hormones progesterone or estrogen are the cause of these breast tumors.

A pathologist, a medical professional who specializes in examining blood and body tissue, can tell if your cancer is ER-positive or PR-positive by examining a sample of your cancer cells to check for the presence of estrogen or progesterone receptors.

In the case of breast cancer, hormone treatment can:

1. Stop cancer from returning.
2. Reduce the likelihood that cancer may spread to other breast tissue.
3. Slow down or stop the spread of cancer.
4. Reduce a tumor's growth before surgery.

Risks

The following are side effects of hormone treatment for breast cancer:

1. Hot flashes.
2. Vaginal discharge.
3. Dryness or irritation of the vagina.
4. Fatigue and Nausea.
5. Muscle and joint discomfort.

The following are less frequent but more severe adverse effects of hormone therapy:

1. veins clogged with blood.
2. Uterine cancer or endometrial cancer.
3. Cataracts.
4. Osteoporosis.

5. Heart condition.
6. Stroke.

Results

While receiving hormone treatment for breast cancer, you will frequently schedule follow-up appointments with your oncologist.

If you are suffering any adverse symptoms, your oncologist will inquire. Many adverse effects are controllable.

In patients with early-stage hormone-sensitive breast cancers, hormone treatment after surgery, radiation, or chemotherapy has been demonstrated to lower the chance of breast cancer recurrence.

It can also successfully lower the chance of developing and spreading hormone-sensitive breast cancers in persons with the disease.

Depending on your scenario, you may be subjected to tests to keep an eye on your health and look for cancer development or recurrence while receiving hormone treatment.

Your doctor can change your therapy based on the results of these tests to gauge how you are reacting to hormone therapy.

CHAPTER SIX

NEED-TO-KNOW ABOUT BREAST CANCER RECURRENCE

Breast cancer that has returned after therapy or after a time when it was undetectable is referred to as a recurrence.

Even after the primary breast cancer has been treated, recurrence might occur months or even years later.

The surgeon removes all of cancer that is visible and palpable during the procedure to remove the primary breast cancer.

However, cancer screening techniques are not sensitive enough to find isolated cancer cells or clusters of a few cancer cells that could survive the surgery.

A tiny number of cells may endure chemotherapy and radiation treatment following surgery.

Any cancer cell that is still present after therapy has been administered may continue to divide and develop into a tumor.

When cancer is discovered in the opposite breast but not elsewhere in the body, it is most likely a new malignancy, not a recurrence.

Local Recurrence

Local recurrence is the term used to describe cancer returning to the same breast or the surgical scar.

Local recurrence symptoms
Similar to those of invasive ductal carcinoma, local recurrence symptoms include:

1. A brand-new breast or chest wall bulge.

2. A breast region where the firmness seems odd.

3. Swelling on some or all breast tissue.

4. Breast-area skin discomfort or redness.

5. Flattening or different nipple alterations.

6. Skin tugging, swelling, or thickening of surgical scars at the location of the first breast cancer surgery.

The breast region may remain swollen and red for a few months following radiation therapy and surgery for breast cancer.

Still, see your doctor if you have any worries about any changes you see in your breasts.

If you had a mastectomy followed by breast reconstruction, you can have lumps brought on by an accumulation of scar tissue or defunct fat cells.

Tell your doctor about any lumps you feel in your breast so they may be checked even if they often aren't cancerous.

Identification of a local recurrence

Several techniques are used to diagnose a local recurrence, and they almost always include:
1. Breast examination
2. Mammogram
3. Biopsy

The following tests may also be used:
1. Ultrasound

2. Breast MRI

Local recurrence Staging
The features of the tumor, such as its size and whether or not it includes hormone receptors, indicate the stage of a local recurrence. You and your doctor can benefit from knowing the recurrent cancer stage:

- Determine your prognosis, or what the disease's likely course will be.

- Choose the most effective course of action for you.

- See if you could be a candidate for certain clinical studies.

The hallmarks of a local recurrence may differ from those of primary breast cancer, according to doctors.

For instance, the local recurrence may be hormone receptor-positive even if the primary tumor was hormone receptor-negative. Your doctor will thus do further tests on the local recurrence. The components of your pathology report include these examinations and the outcomes of your biopsy.

The following details are frequently gathered for a pathology report:
1. The breast cancer size.
2. The cancer stage.
3. Death of the tumor.
4. Cancer margins.
5. Vascular lymph node invasion.
6. Lymph node condition.
7. State of hormone receptors.
8. HER2 status.
9. Cell growth rate (Ki-67 levels).

Care for local recurrence

Treatments for a local recurrence might vary depending on cancer's features and can include:
1. Surgery
2. Radiation treatment

3. Chemotherapy
4. If breast cancer has hormone receptors, hormone treatment may be used.
5. Targeted therapy
6. If the tumor is triple-negative, immunotherapy.

Even so, you and your doctor will consider your prior therapies when deciding on a course of action for the local recurrence if you have previously undergone therapy for breast cancer.

Your doctor will likely advise mastectomy to eliminate the local recurrence if your initial procedure was a lumpectomy.

To address local recurrence, doctors often do not advise a second lumpectomy. When a local recurrence occurs close to the site of a mastectomy, the tumor is often removed if the original surgery was a mastectomy.

Your doctor can advise removing the implant or tissue flap used to reconstruct the breast if the local recurrence occurs in one.

With your medical oncologist and plastic surgeon, you can go through your choices for rebuilding the breast once again.

Your doctor will determine whether radiation therapy is appropriate for the local recurrence if radiation therapy was part of your initial treatment plan based on the location of the local recurrence and the first radiation dosage you received.

Your doctor will take the drugs used into account when determining if chemotherapy, hormonal therapy, targeted therapy, or immunotherapy is appropriate for the local recurrence if any of these treatments were a part of your initial treatment plan.

Regional Recurrence

Regional recurrence denotes the cancer returning to lymph nodes close to the site of the initial diagnosis, such as those in the armpit or collarbone region, the chest wall, or the breast skin.

Signs of a Regional recurrence
The following signs indicate a regional recurrence:
1. Lymph nodes under the arm, above the collarbone, or close to the breastbone that have a lump or swelling.
2. One arm or shoulder may experience pain, swelling, or numbness.
3. Recurring chest pain.

Identification of a Regional recurrence
Several techniques are used to diagnose a local recurrence, and they almost always include:
1. Breast examination

2. Mammogram
3. Biopsy

The following tests may also be used:
1. Ultrasound
2. Breast MRI

Regional recurrence Staging

Regional recurrence is typically regarded as stage III breast cancer and is called locally advanced breast cancer.

Doctors are aware that a localized recurrence of breast cancer may have distinct features from the original disease.

For instance, the localized recurrence may be hormone receptor-positive even if the primary tumor was hormone receptor-negative.

For this reason, your doctor will do further tests on the local recurrence. The components of your pathology report include these examinations and the outcomes of your biopsy.

The following details are frequently gathered for a pathology report:
1. The breast cancer size.
2. The cancer stage.
3. Death of the tumor.
4. Cancer margins.
5. Vascular lymph node invasion.
6. Lymph node condition.
7. State of hormone receptors.
8. HER2 status.
9. Cell growth rate (Ki-67 levels).

Care for Regional recurrence
Treatments for a local recurrence might vary depending on cancer's features and can include:
1. Surgery
2. Radiation treatment
3. Chemotherapy

4. If breast cancer has hormone receptors, hormone treatment may be used.
5. Targeted therapy
6. If the tumor is triple-negative, immunotherapy.

However, because you've already undergone treatment for breast cancer, you and your doctor will take those experiences into account when coming up with a plan of action for the regional recurrence.

Your doctor will probably advise surgery to remove the affected lymph nodes if the regional recurrence affects the armpit or collarbone lymph nodes.

Your doctor will determine whether radiation therapy is appropriate for the regional recurrence if radiation therapy was a component of your initial treatment plan based on the location of the regional recurrence and the initial radiation dose you received.

Your doctor will take the drugs used into account when determining whether chemotherapy, hormonal therapy, targeted therapy, or immunotherapy is appropriate for the regional recurrence if any of these treatments were a part of your initial treatment plan.

Metastatic or Distant Recurrence: Cancer returned in a portion of the body other than the breast, such as the liver, bones, or brain.

CHAPTER SEVEN
LIFE AFTER BREAST CANCER

It's an incredible feeling to receive the "all-clear" diagnosis after receiving a breast cancer diagnosis. However, getting over cancer is a process that takes time. The emotional and physical healing for many women with early-stage breast cancer doesn't start until after the course of treatment is complete.

These suggestions can aid you in navigating the process if you or a loved one is adjusting to life after breast cancer.

Possess reasonable expectations.
Cancer survivors (and their families) may anticipate continuing their lives exactly where they left off after treatment. When treatment ends, depression and anxiety are frequently experienced. People frequently struggle with body image concerns as a

result of scarring, hair loss, and weight fluctuations. Fun? No. Normal. It takes time to feel like yourself again, keep that in mind. In the meanwhile, be kind and patient with yourself (or your loved one). Give yourself the space to reevaluate your requirements as often as necessary—sometimes even every day.

Be fearless.
Patients frequently visit their care team weekly while undergoing therapy. They may then have appointments every three or six months.

Many individuals question whether they are alright. Inform your doctor, nurse, or social worker that you are concerned about speaking with them. T

hey can assist in dispelling rumors and misconceptions and in identifying techniques that give you a sense of more control.

Ensure your wellbeing.
Even if you've heard it before, successful recovery depends on exercise, a balanced diet, sleep, and moderate alcohol use. Exercise is particularly crucial, not just for overall health but also for fighting weariness during recovery.

Demand (Or Offer) Assistance.
During treatment, friends and relatives frequently pitch in by cooking, doing laundry, or picking up the kids from school. That type of helpful assistance frequently ceases abruptly when treatment is completed. The truth is that exhaustion persists even after therapy, especially if you suddenly start working again or adding to your load of home chores. Don't be afraid to seek assistance. Your friends frequently want to support you but are waiting for you to let them know what you require. They may also be unaware that much of the healing process begins after therapy is

completed. And if you're that buddy, find out what you can do to support your loved one as they settle back into their routine.

Speak To Someone Who Understands. Both online and in-person interactions with other survivors can be very beneficial. Connecting through support groups is another excellent option. Finding a group that is facilitated by a qualified professional is key. Not everyone is a good fit for support groups, and that's okay.

On the other hand, I've seen a lot of people who I initially thought didn't belong in support groups give them a shot and benefit greatly from them.

Consider yourself.
Whether it's 5 minutes of deep breathing, 10 minutes of walking outside, or an additional 15 minutes of sleep, do something good for yourself every day. Ask your family for help with whatever it is to make sure it gets done.

Study More.

No matter where they live or receive treatment, Life With Cancer provides free services to cancer patients and their families. In addition to counseling, we also provide art therapy, support groups, fitness classes, mindfulness and meditation, and more.

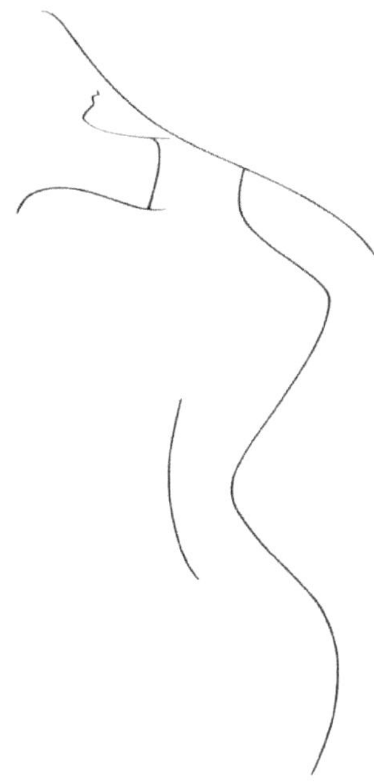

www.ingramcontent.com/pod-product-compliance
Lightning Source LLC
Chambersburg PA
CBHW071223260726

48653CB00042B/1767